20 WAYS TO STAY HEALTHY IN RETIREMENT.

Enjoying optimum health in retirement can be achieved.

By

Dr DOUGLAS JASON

TABLE OF CONTENTS

TABLE OF CONTENTS

ABOUT THE AUTHOR

Dr DOUGLAS JASON is a certified dietician who has a strong passion for wellness and a big eagerness to help people all over the world. He uses healthy food, herbs, sauce and other useful tools to help mankind realized it's overall goal of optimum health.

INTRODUCTION

A key life milestone is a retirement. After years of rigorous effort, now is a time to enjoy and unwind. To get the most out of this stage of life, however, it is essential to retain excellent health after retirement. While aging is a natural process, by taking care of our physical, mental, and emotional health, we may age gracefully. We'll go over some crucial advice for maintaining your health after retirement in this post.

CHAPTER 1

REMAIN ACTIVE IN THE PHYSICAL.

It's crucial to be active to keep your health in excellent shape. Frequent exercise may help maintain a healthy body weight, lower the chance of developing chronic illnesses, and enhance mental health. People tend to become less active after retirement, which may cause several health problems. As a result, it's crucial to maintain your physical fitness by partaking in activities like walking, cycling, swimming, or yoga.

CHAPTER 2

DISCOVER A NEW PURPOSE.

Retirement is more than just leaving your career. Your life transitions into a new phase. You'll be happier and healthier if you engage in meaningful work. Donate your time to a hospital or library. Partake in training at your place of worship. Those who need tutoring should do so. maintenance of refuge for animals. Assemble care packages for troops serving abroad. This has long-term benefits for your health and mind.

CHAPTER 3

Maintain a Balanced Diet.

After retirement, it's critical to maintain excellent health by eating a balanced, wholesome diet. Our bodies need fewer calories as we get older, but we still need the same amount of nutrients. Chronic illnesses may be prevented, the immune system can be strengthened, and general health can be enhanced with a balanced diet high in fruits, vegetables, whole grains, lean protein, and healthy fats.

CHAPTER 4

THE PROPER SURROUNDINGS.

Your health may be better off depending on where you reside. You may choose from a range of options if you desire pure air. You may work out outside while surrounded by the mountains in Boulder, the sea in Portland, Maine, or the sun in Tucson, Arizona. Being close to Cleveland, Boston, Baltimore, Houston, New York City, or Rochester might be advantageous for receiving top-notch medical treatment.

CHAPTER 5

MAN OR WOMAN'S BEST FRIEND

A dog offers you more than just unconditional affection. Spending only 15 minutes with Fido may significantly reduce stress, blood pressure, and heart rate. A devoted friend may eventually aid in lowering cholesterol, combating melancholy, and maintaining your level of activity. Moreover, owning a cat helps reduce stress and blood pressure.

CHAPTER 6

HEALTHY FOOD

As you get older, you're more likely to experience nutrition-related issues like weight loss or vitamin deficiency. A diet rich in protein, fat, and carbohydrates is therefore more crucial than ever. Reduce your intake of packaged foods because they are high in salt and can cause your blood pressure to rise. Eating a lot of fruit, vegetables, whole grains, and olive oil, as is the custom in Greece and the surrounding area, is a good choice.

CHAPTER 7

GET OUT OF THE HOUSE.

Living an active lifestyle can improve your mood, lengthen your life, and reduce your risk of developing certain diseases, such as dementia. Play cards with your buddies. Join a senior citizen tour group. re-establish contact with old high school or college pals. Join a club that specializes in your hobby, such as reading, knitting, or gardening.

CHAPTER 8

Keep tabs on your health.

Frequent medical exams are essential. By keeping an eye on your blood pressure and cholesterol, your doctor can help you prevent a heart attack or a stroke. You can stave against the flu and other infections by getting immunizations on time. You should be checked for breast and cervical cancer if you're a woman, and your doctor may advise you on whether to get checked for prostate cancer if you're a guy.

CHAPTER 9

EXERCISE FOR FUN AND FITNESS.

Staying active helps you maintain your independence as you age in addition to improving your health. Choose an enjoyable activity so you will continue doing it. Walking, swimming, or dancing are all aerobic exercises that may help you feel more energized and keep your mind sharp. Strengthening exercises may be done using bands or weights. Yoga makes you more flexible. If you've never exercised before, start slowly and see your doctor first.

CHAPTER 10

BEHIND THE WHEEL.

The ability to drive safely may be impacted by changes in your vision, physical condition, and reflexes throughout time. Keeping tabs is essential for your protection. Can you notice the road signs? Are you mobile enough to reverse your automobile and check for oncoming traffic? Do you get confused by traffic? With problems like these, your doctor may be able to assist. Also, organizations like AARP and AAA provide workshops to help you assess and improve your abilities.

CHAPTER 11

BONE HEALTH

Women need to strengthen their bones. Osteoporosis is a disorder where your bones become more brittle due to hormonal changes that occur after menopause. Make sure your food provides you with enough calcium, the main component of bones, to combat that. Broccoli, spinach, nonfat or low-fat milk, and yogurt are all excellent sources. Have a low-dose X-ray called a DEXA test performed on your bones by your doctor when you turn 65.

CHAPTER 12

SOCIALIZE AND CONNECT.

The impact of social isolation on one's physical and mental health can be detrimental. Many people may experience despair and anxiety after retiring, as a result of feeling alone. To maintain social ties and mental health, it is essential to stay in touch with family and friends, join social clubs or groups, or volunteer.

CHAPTER 13

STIMULATE YOUR MIND

Like your body, your mind needs a workout. Take up a new activity, read, solve puzzles, play an instrument, or do any of the above. Enroll in a class on a topic you're interested in, such as computers or food. Also, exercising your creative side through hobbies like painting and gardening can support brain health. For instance, taking an acting class could improve your memory and problem-solving abilities.

CHAPTER 14

ASK FOR YOUR 40 WINKS.

As you get older, it could be more difficult for you to sleep through the night. To relieve joint pain, you might need to urinate or adjust your position in bed. But you can help by taking action. 2 hours before bedtime, stop consuming liquids. Avoid caffeine for eight hours before bed. Darken the space as much as you can. Limit naps during the day to 10 or 20 minutes. Ask your doctor if you should take a pain reliever before bed to aid with aches.

CHAPTER 15

SAFETY AROUND THE HOUSE

As you age, mishaps in the home become riskier. Get non-slip mats for the tub and bathroom floor. Repair carpets or rugs that are frayed. Make sure there is enough light. Secure any dangling cords. Install handrails on both sides of any stairs in your home, and add anti-slip strips to the steps themselves.

CHAPTER 16:

SLEEP ENOUGH.

Especially after retirement, getting adequate sleep is essential for maintaining good health. Several factors, including prescription drugs and medical issues, might make it difficult for older folks to fall asleep. To encourage sound sleeping habits, it is crucial to create a regular sleep schedule, unwind before bed, and stay away from caffeine and alcohol.

Chapter 17

Impacies

Sexuality may disappear from your life due to physical changes. But, you may restore the sizzle. Each of you should first express your thoughts and worries to the other. Assure your partner that you still find them attractive. Massages and holding hands are effective methods for reuniting. See your doctor if there is a physical issue, such as erectile dysfunction.

CHAPTER 18

MANAGE YOUR TIME WELL.

Having time on your hands is one of the key benefits of retirement. You are free to act whenever you like. According to studies, retirees are happiest when they make the most of their time and plan how to spend it. Even if you don't have a lot of free time if you manage it efficiently, that can pay dividends. Also, it can prevent boredom.

CHAPTER 19

Working After Retirement:

Working after retirement can keep your mind and body sharp, not to mention your bank account. Do a more streamlined version of your previous job if you liked it. It is a choice for occupations including bookkeeping, home health care, and home repair. Or perhaps this is your time to try out the job you've always been interested in. The most satisfying careers are occasionally second ones.

CHAPTER 20

REGULAR HEALTH CHECK-UPS

After retirement, maintaining excellent health requires routine medical exams. Many health problems brought on by aging can be prevented by early detection and treatment. Frequent health examinations can aid in the early detection of conditions like high blood pressure, diabetes, or cancer and enable prompt action.

CONCLUSION.

After retirement, maintaining good health is crucial to living a happy life. Maintaining a healthy lifestyle and avoiding chronic diseases can be achieved by participating in physical activity, eating a balanced diet, keeping up with friends and family, getting adequate sleep, and scheduling routine medical exams. Our bodies change as we get older, and so do our health requirements. To age gracefully, it is necessary to adjust to these changes and to take good care of our physical, mental, and emotional health.